The smart way to lose weight quickly:

Simple Solutions for Typical Weight Loss Challenges

Betty D. Rivera

Table of contents

Chapter 1

How to Surmount Typical Obstacles to Weight Loss

If you have struggled to lose weight, you are not alone. Everybody has different challenges while trying to lose weight. Healthy weight reduction may be hampered by factors such as your body image, genetics, life circumstances, stress, money, time, and time limits, but that doesn't mean you can't make an effort to overcome them.

Most people should prepare themselves for challenges along the route to their weight loss goals. Learning to tackle weight loss challenges when they arise is key to losing weight and keeping it off.

Identifying Weight Loss Barriers
One must first search within to start. Several of the challenges you are facing have previously

been overcome, so keep that in mind. Maintaining a healthy diet and exercise routine is not always easy. The majority of people have ups and downs in life. Once you've identified your obstacles, you may work on developing the skills necessary to get through them.

Some barriers to weight loss are perceived barriers, which means that your thoughts or emotions are to blame. Perceived barriers can be just as significant and real as actual ones, and examples include physical limitations and adverse health conditions. Depending on whether they are imagined or real, your difficulties can be categorized into three fundamental categories: physical, environmental, and emotional.

Physical Barriers to Weight Loss
Physical barriers to weight loss typically include fatigue, discomfort, and underlying medical issues. Your capacity to shed weight may also be impacted by dehydration and sleep deprivation. Despite the sizeableness of these challenges,

there are ways to get around them and still lose weight.

Communication With Your Doctor
Consult your doctor about your weight loss concerns. Perhaps a health issue is the root of your annoyance.

For instance, several medications (including steroid medications, birth control pills, and some antidepressants) may cause weight gain. If you just gave up smoking, you might gain weight.

Physical Barriers to Weight Loss
Physical barriers to weight loss typically include fatigue, discomfort, and underlying medical issues. Your capacity to shed weight may also be impacted by dehydration and sleep deprivation. Despite the sizeableness of these challenges, there are ways to get around them and still lose weight.

Hormonal changes, such as those brought on by menopause, might make it more difficult to reduce weight and encourage weight gain. Medical conditions include PCOS and a few thyroid diseases are associated with weight gain.

Improve Your Sleep
Scientists have discovered that gastrointestinal problems can result from insufficient sleep. When you don't receive the rest you need, your hormonal balance may change, and you may experience increased hunger and appetite. Evidence suggests that people who receive shorter, more frequent periods of sleep (under seven hours) are more likely to be overweight or obese.

Fortunately, implementing a few changes to your sleep schedule may help you achieve your weight loss goals. To promote a relaxing environment, experts advise that you fall asleep at the same time every night, sleep in a cool, dark room, and turn off any electronic devices (such as tablets and cellphones).

Get some water

Making small adjustments to your daily routine can make losing weight easier. One simple change that has numerous medicinal benefits is staying hydrated. More water consumption is associated with improved weight loss outcomes, according to studies.

Being confused by the signals of hunger and thirst is quite normal. To get in and out of your refrigerator, keep filled water bottles there. If you want enhanced drinks, consider adding berries or other ingredients (such as basil or cucumber). If you find yourself brushing in the kitchen throughout the day, consider sipping a few ounces of water before a meal to see if it satisfies your craving.

Create Calorie-Efficient Recipes for Enhanced Water

Complete Your Work.

Examine several schedules for activities and reliable cooking advice. When they're amusing, behaviors that result in weight loss are more rational. For instance, if you suffer from weight, pain, or joint problems, non-weight-bearing workouts like water high-impact exercise may be more tolerable.

Change your regular dinner routine by enrolling in a practical cooking class. You'll learn better ways to prepare vegetables or lean meats and enjoy your time in the kitchen.

Environmental Barriers to Weight Loss
It can feel like a waste of time and energy when your surroundings don't support a healthy food regimen and exercise routine. Natural barriers might make losing weight seem impossible, such as access restrictions to healthy food or exercise facilities, poor social support, or a lack of time due to interpersonal, familial, or professional conflicts.

Talk to People Around You Share Your Needs to Gain Support from Family and Friends Be clear about how they can help make your agreement successful. Perhaps your partner will run extra errands, or your kids will pitch in more around the house.

Your boss might support your healthy lifestyle by providing resources for your well-being or flexibility in your work-related plans. A more effective representative makes a better employee. Fortunately, more and more companies are beginning to see the benefits of health programs.

Get Creative and Workout
Numerous options for at-home fitness are available if traveling to the gym is not an option for you. On the web, there are free workouts available (really take a look at YouTube or Instagram). There are also a ton of mobile and tablet applications that offer programming practice. You can find a variety of classes as well as hints, conversations, and other resources.

You can also use the resources right outside your door to improve your health. Walking is an excellent kind of exercise. Take a stroll through your neighborhood, ascend the stairs in your building or complex, or organize family climbs over the weekend. Many malls provide special hours for walkers who need to hone their skills before the groups take over.

Boundaries to weight loss that are nearby
It sounds absurd to claim that you need to lose weight, but your feelings about it are keeping you down. However, local barriers to weight loss are undeniable and frequently significant. These obstacles may include doubts about your ability to accomplish your goals, a poor relationship with your actual work, intense worry, or just a lack of motivation.

Enlist a Certified Expert's Assistance
Many people with conduct wellness training, like social workers, consultants, and therapists, focus on the emotions related to body weight. If you have proactively looked into potential medical explanations for your weight problems, you might want to talk to a professional about more serious concerns.

Learn How to Motivate Yourself
You can become an inspiration expert. It has been shown that techniques like journaling and positive self-talk can boost your inspiration and propel you in the right direction.

Additionally, self-observation is an effective tool for weight loss.

Maintaining a food journal, regularly monitoring your weight, or tracking your actual work with a paper log or an app are all examples of self-checking. Self-checking helps you become aware of your regular behaviors so you can develop the focus necessary to make changes as needed.

Step-by-step Guidelines to Motivate Yourself to Lose Weight
Utilize pressure reduction techniques
Stress can quickly lead to binge eating and weight gain if it is related to your hectic schedule, family problems, an inability to lose

weight, or a chronic illness. Obesity and constant pressure are connected.

However, techniques for reducing stress (such as deep breathing or focused perception) have been shown to improve weight loss results.

Learn techniques for reducing pressure, such as deep breathing, contemplation, or journaling. Schedule these workouts throughout your day to put yourself in the best frame of mind for growth.

Boundaries to weight loss that are nearby

Remember that reaching and maintaining a healthy weight is a long race, not a sprint. Similar to how one day of prudent diets won't make up for a month of poor choices, the contrary is also clear.

Utilize the opportunities you have in your daily life to make healthy choices. Feeling your best at any weight can be achieved by balancing your style of life with regular vigorous work and stress.

Chapter 2

The Right Hunger Levels To Achieve When Trying To Lose Weight

Not continuously feeling hungry is the secret to weight loss. It might seem like a necessary evil that weight loss causes constant hunger. You can anticipate dealing with cravings all day long because you're consuming fewer calories. Wait a second. That doesn't just sound like a miserable way to live; it also won't help you in your weight-loss attempts. Even worse, it might work against you.

Overeating can make unhealthy foods more enticing, make you feel too weak to give your best during exercise, and if you don't consume enough calories, it can even stop you from losing weight.

Here's how to tell if the discomfort you're experiencing is simply a normal part of life or whether it's leading you astray.

First of all, accept the fact that while you will undoubtedly be hungry, you shouldn't always be so.

The majority of experts advise eating regularly whether or not you're trying to get fitter. That suggests you'll likely experience some degree of hunger daily. "If you're eliminating calories after [being used to] eating a lot of food, you'll probably have some desire, and that's normal, However, if the hunger is constant, distracting, and you can see that it's causing you to overeat or make poor choices when you were last eating, then you probably need to eat more.

Identify how to decide just how ravenous you genuinely are after that, and determine your ideal equilibrium.

Reco considers the predisposition to rate your desire on a scale of one to ten. A five to seven on this scale represents the longing for perfect balance, while a one indicates that you are typically completely satisfied. A 10 indicates that you need to rip off your arm and eat it to satisfy yourself. When you consume a meal or a snack, you should be in that position. She explains, "On the odd chance that you're experiencing something between an eight and a ten, you'll indulge." You can control how much food you eat while you're between the ages of five and seven, according to the scale.

A word of caution: sometimes the craving you're experiencing isn't even related to hunger. "Our bodies frequently decipher thirst as hunger, so we'll feel hungry even though we're simply parched," says Dr. "Drink some water, wait 10 to 20 minutes, and see whether the 'hunger' goes away," "You're not kidding, assuming it's still there," she said. In addition, stress and fatigue regularly cause people to reach for a beverage when their bodies don't need sustenance.

Additionally, if you're just starting on your weight loss journey, your former eating schedule may somewhat confuse the indications. If you're used to mindlessly nibbling throughout the day (which can unintentionally result in excessive calorie intake), you might feel mentally "hungry" because you miss the habit. The longer you stick to this new smart dieting plan, the better your body will adapt to less nibbling throughout the day.

There are techniques to look into the problem if you have abnormal amounts of appetite throughout the day.

Denying oneself isn't ideal, either conceptually or authentically. Make sure you are consuming the calories you desire if, despite eating, you continue to feel as though you have an appetite of an 8, 9, or 10. Make a point to determine whether you're consuming enough calories to lose weight.

Next, look into the presentation of your feasts. "Do all of your dinners contain high-quality protein, such as beans, eggs, Greek yogurt, tofu, beef, and fish? Is it accurate to suggest that you consume a lot of vegetables? Is it safe to assume that you have completely cut back on sugar? Don't worry that eating carbs like whole wheat bread will interfere with your attempts to lose weight; in certain circumstances, consuming a small number of carbs at a feast helps you feel satisfied. Due to their filling fiber, complex carbohydrates can significantly help you lose weight.

It can also help with planning when you become envious by finding designs (keeping an everyday food log might assist with this). If you have no stomach issues during the day but do so every night before bed, the following plausible circumstances and logical outcomes are probably at work: It makes sense that your body would become somewhat boisterous when you train yourself to eat every three to four hours, eat at night, and stay up late. If this is a concern of yours, you should probably go to bed earlier. This can be challenging, but it's probably a good idea if you're trying to lose weight.

It's best to sleep off, then wake up and eat a lot of protein-rich dinners and snacks to avoid having a similar inclination the next day, assuming it's right before bed and you know you've eaten enough and are going to go to sleep. Don't torture yourself to lose weight, though, if all you're thinking about is the large opening in your stomach and you're only going to eat a little. Your goals won't be derailed by one tidbit! Have a sensible snack, go to bed, and don't worry about it.

Chapter 3

How To Lose Weight Easily, Permanently, And Normally

When you're bombarded with advice like eating wholesome meals and leading a healthy lifestyle, it can be challenging for many people to lose weight. Even the use of diet pills is being promoted by some people. You regularly check your progress in the mirror, but there are no changes there despite your efforts to lose weight. A little progress is visible, but then the weight gain flare-ups return.

I've included steps you can take to help you get in shape naturally, so don't worry. I have included information on how to lose weight effectively and keep it off if you find that you can't keep up with all you need to lose.

While losing weight naturally can be difficult, you might be more motivated if you believe that super long-lasting weight loss is possible. This is how to get slimmer routinely and stay up with it because we are getting right to it.

Enhancements to a typical fat burner
If you're looking for a reliable, effective, and safe weight-loss solution, go no further than fat-killer supplements. Fat terminators are substances that help you lose weight more quickly by enhancing digestion and reducing hunger. They are made with potent ingredients like caffeine and green tea concentrate. Make sure to heed the name's cues and accept it as coordinated if you want to profit from your fat-burning pill.

Consume only one type of food at a time.
Do you consume a daily amount of sugar? You are already attempting to avoid consuming fat and added sugar from processed food when you eat whole, single-fixing food variety. In addition to providing your body with essential supplements, it can keep you full for a long time.

Refrain from consuming any type of handled food.

The sugar, fats, and calories in these meal types are frequently high. Additionally, the purpose of these food sources is to encourage you to consume more than is reasonable.

Hold a supply of wholesome foods and reliable snacks.

According to a study, your eating habits are influenced by the food sources you have at home, which also affects your attempts to lose weight. You are more likely to eat high-quality food if you have a good selection of foods. You are more likely to consume unhealthy meals if you consume low-quality food. There are numerous options for high-quality foods, including whole organic products, veggies, almonds, and hard-boiled eggs.

Include protein

According to Wellbeing Waterway Magazine, when it comes to weight loss, protein is regarded as the king of supplements. The body is using calories in addition to proteins at this time as it processes them. The digestion is therefore aided, resulting in a daily calorie reduction of 80–100. Hunger and cravings are also reduced.

Absent added sugar at any costs
Type 2 diabetes can be brought on by consuming sweet food sources, especially processed ones where fake sugars are added, which can increase your blood glucose levels. The most terrifying aspect of all is that food markings are frequently absent. You won't lose weight, and you might even gain weight if you try it.

Hydrate Water has a part in weight loss, especially if you drink it in place of calorie- and sugar-rich beverages. 24–30% of the calories in 0.5 liters of water are destroyed. Additionally, reducing calorie intake is drinking water before meals.

Coffee without sugar Actually, coffee includes chemicals that fight cancer and may increase digestion by 3–11%. Although it almost entirely lacks calories, it simultaneously increases your energy and cheers you on.

Keep fluid calories to a minimum
Commercial organic product juices, pop cans, and caffeinated beverages are a few examples of fluid calories. It doesn't help with weighing bad luck but instead increases the chance of becoming strong all else being equal.

Limit refined carbohydrates.

These are food sources that also include considerable amounts of fiber and other nutrients, yet all that is left are carbohydrates. You will frequently consume more than you should because these are not food types that require much processing. White bread and white rice are two examples of refined sugars. Given everything, you could substitute it with rice that is earthy in hue.

Fasting Occasionally

It is a practice of eating and fasting that involves food. It can be done in a variety of ways, but it generally helps you consume fewer calories.

Eat more leafy foods

These nutrient-dense food types also include water and other additives and are high in fiber. Since they don't contain a lot of energy, even if you eat a lot of them, you won't necessarily consume too many calories.

Diet Low In Carbs

Your appetite also declines when you consume fewer carbohydrates and more proteins. This is even significantly more effective than a typical low-fat eating plan, according to a study, by numerous orders of magnitude.

Calories in.

A good way to reduce the number of calories you eat each day is to actively keep track of what you eat and how much you consume.

Calorie restriction has been mentioned earlier as a weight-loss strategy.

Eating Slowly

Don't eat too quickly because your body might later realize that you are full. So, you'll consume more calories than you anticipated. While this is happening, eating more slowly helps your body produce more hormones linked to weight loss.

Steer clear of sleep deprivation

Lack of sleep disrupts the changes in hunger-related hormones, which leads to undesirable desire patterns. People who have trouble sleeping tend to be heavier.

Take in More Fiber

Fiber makes a significant contribution to efficient processing. It can also provide you with a few hours of encouragement while improving your digestion. To change your fiber intake, combine whole grains and refined grains with meals that are cultivated from the ground.

Blocking Behaviors

Not only does it help you lose weight, but it also prevents a lack of mass. People who lack mass frequently end up gaining weight again. However, it differs somewhat from obstructive techniques like weightlifting.

Aware Eating

This is a potent technique for overcoming intense eating or eating under stress. It increases your awareness of what you consume so that you can decide whether to restrict your calorie intake or avoid foods high in calories.

Is it Possible to Lose 10 Pounds in a Week?

Some people can lose 10 pounds in just seven days. However, experts in the field concur that not everyone can make it happen. Certainly, if you try to handle it by yourself, you might put yourself in risky situations. Getting monitored by your doctor is great if it is not necessary to achieve such a purpose.

Being thinner forever can be a problem from the start. In any event, we offer a ton of strategies for losing weight that can help you reach your goal. You wouldn't always be aware of how to become fitter while also being aware of how to regularly get in shape.